I Am
NOT
Cancer

*How I Was Able to Stay Calmer
Through My Cancer Journey
and You Can Too*

Carol L Rickard, LCSW

Stage III Cancer Survivor
America's Ultimate Stress Expert

**WellYOUniversity®
Publications**

I Am NOT Cancer
by Carol L Rickard, LCSW

Published by Well YOUniversity® Publications. Well YOUniversity® is a registered trademark of Well YOUniversity, LLC.

ISBN: 978-1-947745-30-8 (paperback)
ISBN: 978-1-947745-35-3 (Ebook)

Don't Miss Out...

> ## A Special Gift
>
> ## Is Waiting
>
> ## Just For You!

Carol has put together a
special eBook just for you...

To sign up for
"Your C.A.L.M. Toolbox"

Go to:

StandTallToCancer.com

I Am NOT Cancer

An easy user-friendly book to help those unwell, improve their mindset so they can carry on their journey better enabled to fight their battles. Recommended for children and adults.

- Helen Szoke, RN

Carol knocks it out of the park again! Another thoughtful, personal, and practical book to get us through the challenges of life. Although not a cancer survivor, I found the exercises helpful with a different health challenge I am undergoing. I find the exercises help me to get moving when I feel emotionally stuck in an unhelpful place. Thank You Carol for using your own difficult experience to help others......

- Pat Brennan LCSW

I have loved all of Carol's books, both in their content and the way they are presented. However, this one is my absolute favorite! Carol's authenticity and vulnerability in sharing her personal journey gives so much power and credibility to the effectiveness of the stress tools, and how they work in one of life's biggest challenges. Her sincere desire to help other people with cancer navigate the process is palpable. This book is truly a gift of love.

- Shirley Roberts, MA, LPC, NCC

Praise For I Am NOT Cancer

"I Am Not Cancer" offers insight regarding the importance of mindset and how to overcome stress. This focus allows YOU to have control. The variety of tools Carol has offered are do-able and effective.

As a survivor, I agree that we are not cancer. May the information in this book provide you with motivation, new information and hope on your journey.

- Sheila Riley-Massa, MPA, MT-BC

A powerful and essential book for anyone who feels they are battling their cancer.

- Daniel Herrera, Founder Communify

It is my goal to "love health" more than "battle cancer". Peace cannot be had with war. This book is all about creating health and peace within me. I know I am surviving stage 4 metastasized breast cancer because of my shift of thoughts. Anyone can benefit from Carol's book, but especially those creating health around cancer. Thank you for affirming my idea, in writing.

- Shari Viger, Stage 4 Cancer Thriver

Table of Contents

Introduction

Part One: The Foundation

Part Two: Taking Control of Stress

Addendum

My Starting Point

As I sat in the treatment room waiting for my doctor to come in, it felt like I'd been waiting for over an hour. But it was only 15 minutes before the door opened and she walked in.

I'd been to see her the week before, for a procedure. At that time, she thought there was an issue with my estrogen levels and had given me some information to look over about different medications I could try. I was seeing her today to discuss which one I'd chosen.

As she began to speak, I was completely blindsided…

"Carol it's cancer."

I quickly had this thought: *'Well, it could be worse. It could have been there, and I never knew it. At least now I can do something about it.'* And immediately I felt a wave of gratitude come over me.

And so, my cancer journey began.

As I drove home from the doctor's office, I found myself thinking God was giving me a new assignment. You see I'd spent 30 years teaching patients in hospitals how to better manage stress.

And the way I saw it, the only way I could ever truly help a cancer patient learn to better manage stress was to go through that experience myself. And so, I did.

Which brings me to today...

This book is written to help me fulfill part of that assignment from God! I'm going to share with you exactly what I did to take control of the incredible stress that comes along with a cancer diagnosis & stay calmer so you can too.

It doesn't matter whether you're the person with cancer, a family member, a friend, or even a healthcare practitioner... *Cancer stress is a part of your life.*

It also doesn't matter whether you have chosen a traditional treatment route or an alternative one. **The stress is there.**

What You Will Learn

There are four critical lessons you will walk away with from this book:

1) *The mindset* you MUST have to successfully navigate your cancer journey.

2) Learning why *stress management* is not enough & how Rapid Relief Therapy™ can put you back in charge.

3) Understanding WHY you *must take action* to deal with stress.

4) A simple & practical system that can *reduce CANCER STRESS & ANXIETY* levels in just 60 seconds or less.

My bold promise to you is this:

This book will help you take control of cancer stress and anxiety to stay calmer through your cancer journey. However, you need to realize it's not a magic pill... It will only help if you take action and use what you're about to learn!

Using This Book

This book is divided in to two parts. **Part One** is focused on building a foundation for your success and that begins with what I call *The Survivor's Mindset.* You'll learn what and why a "mindset" is an important piece of recovery.

You'll also learn the four cornerstones of my recovery, that when put together with Part Two of this book, provide a rock-solid foundation for success.

Part Two is designed to be more like a mini workshop in a book! You'll learn the exact blueprint and tools I used every day since my diagnosis to stay in control of stress & anxiety and stay calmer through my cancer journey.

Presented in a little different format, Part Two is based on my 30 years of experience teaching people life changing skills. It is more of a "visual" experience. I like to use a lot of pictures, analogies, and word art which help the information stick in the brain.

Part One

The Foundation

The Survivor's Mindset

One of the first and most valuable cancer lessons I learned came from colleagues who I refer to as my "Guardian Angels". These were two women, both of whom I had a tremendous amount of professional respect for and who were 20-year breast cancer survivors. They both told me the same thing:

"Carol – it's all about your mindset."

I also had two other friends in my life, additional "Guardian Angels" who influenced my **Survivor Mindset™**. Both were friends who'd battled with terminal illnesses other than cancer.

I'd met Alicia a year earlier and we got to become friends when I helped her publish her memoir. Not only is she a 14-year survivor of Stage 3 Melanoma, but she also had an incredible recovery from the deadly Steven Johnsons Disease. Reading her story, "The Miracle of Me". is one of the most inspiring stories I'd ever experienced and a great example of '**_Survivor Mindset_**' in action.

The other friend, Hope Taylor, had been in my life for over 20 years. The way she lived her life despite having Lupus for 35+ years taught me so much. Hope had the type of Lupus which is terminal as it slowly attacks all the organs in the body and there are no cures for it.

But you'd have never known that by the way she lived her life... Lupus was NOT going to define her life for her – she was! (It was during a moment when I was writing to her in my Honor Book I'd created after her passing in Nov. 2020 that the idea and title for this book came to me.)

Shortly after my diagnosis I realized that despite my experience working in healthcare for so long, I really didn't know much about cancer other than the fact that both my parents died from it. I decided I needed to learn more since I was going to need to be making decisions about it.

** I believe this is a critical step people often fail to do. Please DO NOT rely solely on your doctor to educate you on all there is to know about your cancer – educate yourself!

The first book I read and highly recommend – whether you are the patient or the family member - is Dr. Kelly Turner's "Radical Remission". Now I'm not just saying that because she's a fellow social worker!

The book is filled with powerful stories of people who were told they had terminal cancer or there was nothing more that could be done for them, only to be alive 10, 15, 20 years later! It included people who used both traditional and alternative approaches. What I love most is that Dr. Turner helps us see how the prevailing mindset around cancer: cancer diagnosis = death, is not so true! The reader walks away with the true beginnings of "*Survivor Mindset*".

I ended up reading many great books that spoke to the *Survivor Mindset™*. Please check out a list of them in the resources section at the back of this book.

What Is Mindset?

So, you may be wondering, what is a mindset? According to Merriam Webster, mindset is:

1) A mental attitude or inclination
2) A fixed state of mind

A simple definition I've given my patients over the years is:

⇒ The way we *think* about things

A*ll of us* have mindset, though most people aren't even aware that they do! It runs silently in the background of our brain, influencing everything in our lives.

In fact, we have many different mindsets: you have your money mindset, your relationship mindset, your spiritual mindset, etc. Well, you get the point! They all influence the many different areas of our lives.

An analogy I like to use is that mindset is like the operating system of a computer. The OS or operating system of a computer is what allows us to have all the different software and hardware we like to use. It basically "runs" the computer! And our mindsets basically "run" our lives!

One of the earliest lessons I learned about mindset happened my first day on the job in December of 1991 when I started working as a Recreation Therapist on a mental health / addiction treatment unit.

I was sitting in on a therapy group when the doctor said to a patient: *"You are NOT your addiction. You are a person who is living with an addiction."* This mindset, that **who I am is not based on the circumstances of my life**, has remained with me ever since then. And it has been a cornerstone of my cancer recovery: **I am not cancer!**

In the next sections, I'm going to share with you the 4 cornerstones of my *Survivor Mindset™*: Gratitude, Wellness, Healing., and Acceptance.

The Gratitude Switch
Cornerstone #1

The first cornerstone has to do with our brain and the amazing power it holds! What most people don't realize is they can control how that power is used to influence their lives! All it takes is a bit of "Brain Training".

One of the ways I've trained my brain is to make gratitude be the first thought response when something happens in my life. The good news is you can too!

First, I want to help you understand why "Brain Training" is an important thing to do. Our brain has all this incredible power that can either HELP us or HURT us. We can control which one of those it does! Here's an example:

Have you ever tried to reach a family member by phone and after many tries of not being able to reach them you suddenly had this thought?

'Oh my God, what if they were in an accident or are lying in a hospital somewhere?'

I used to have this exact thought! And what's worse, the thought would cause a feeling - panic - which then caused me to be physically sick to my stomach! All within a split second.

Once I learned about 'Brain Training' I was able to have a different response when the same type of situation would happen...

'Well maybe they're just super busy or maybe they've gone out of town and don't get very good cell reception.'

Can you see how this thought would cause me to remain calm?

So, how do you do "Brain Training"?

Well, there are so *many* different types of exercises & activities you can do. And we'll get in to some more of them later in this book. But since we're kind of limited in space, if you really want to take your "Brain Training" to a whole new level, then you may want to check out one of my online classes or attend a live workshop where that is all that we focus on! That's why you want to make sure you're on our mailing list to get notices of upcoming classes & workshops.

Did you know that according to research by the National Science Foundation, your brain averages 12,000 to 60,000 **thoughts** per **day**? Of those, 80% **are negative** and 95% are repetitive **thoughts**.

So, when my patients used to say their goal was to "not think negative" I'd have to make them change their goal... It is impossible to not THINK NEGATIVE! Instead, what we must do is train our brain to *ignore the negative* and **FOCUS on the positive!** This is what "Brain Training" helps us do!

The exercise I want to share with you right now is one you can use to train your brain to think *gratitude* as your thought response. I call it **"The Gratitude Switch™"**.

Here's how it goes:

Step 1: The next time anything happens in your life, I want you to finish the sentence below by identifying at least one way the situation could be worse.

> *"It could be worse,......it (or) I could have* [identify & state a worse outcome]."

Step 2: You must say the whole sentence out loud. Don't just say it in your head!

Here's just a few of my real-life examples:

Running 15 minutes late for work - *"It could be worse; I could have been an hour late."*

Car accident – *"It could be worse; I could have been hurt or even killed."*

Cancer Diagnosis – *"It could be worse; it could have been there, and I never knew it.*

It may seem like hard work at first. But I promise you, "Brain Training" is just like any other type of training: the more consistent you are doing it, the better you get at it and the easier it becomes! Keep practicing!!!

Bonus Tip:

Look for ways to practice this throughout your day using the everyday small stuff stressing you out: kids running late, traffic, getting ready for work or school, etc.... You wouldn't wait to practice your swimming skills until you needed them on the Titanic, would you?

Destination: Wellness
Cornerstone #2

This brings us to the 2nd cornerstone of my *Survivor Mindset™* which is **Wellness.**

Every moment of every day we have a choice to make: We either focus on wellness or focus on illness. What we can't do is focus on both at the same time.

Imagine for a moment you're driving a car. You can only move it one of two directions – either forward or backward. It is impossible for it to do both at the same time!

Our brain works the same way in that it can only truly focus on one thought at a time. This is why the **Gratitude Switch™** works so well because the brain cannot focus on a negative and positive thought at the same time! We're "choosing" a positive thought to focus on.

To help you better understand this, I have a little experiment I'd like you to try that I learned from Dean Graziosi and it will only take a minute to do.

First, I want you to think about the Statue of Liberty for a moment. Picture it in your mind. Can you see it? Next, I want you to think about the Grand Canyon for a moment. Picture it in your mind. Can you see it? Now, I want you to think about BOTH at the same time for a moment. Can you picture it in your mind?

No, you can't because it is simply impossible! Our brain cannot focus on two different thoughts at the same time. Likewise, our brains cannot focus on wellness & getting better when we are so busy talking and thinking about our cancer (the illness).

The tool I want to share with you right now is one I use to train my brain to stay focused on *wellness* and how you can too. I call it "**Ticket to Wellness!™**".

I first came up with this idea 30 years ago during my work as a Recreation Therapist. I'd have my patients make a key chain to take home with them that would be a good reminder of WHY they were wanting to stay sober and well.

I wanted to create a visible reminder of that reason. So, when their brain was flooded with all the other stress and happenings in their world, they had an "anchor" to keep them focused on what was most important in their life: sobriety. Because without that – they wouldn't have anything else.

When the cancer diagnosis showed up in my life and my brain was flooded with all the stress and decisions that needed to be made, I realized I needed an "anchor" to keep me focused on what was most important to me: getting well!

So, I created my **Ticket to Wellness™,** and I carried it on me everywhere I went, and I would look at it often to keep me focused on wellness. Again, it's training the brain!

Here's what to do:

Step 1: Identify something you want to *do or have happen* in your life more than anything else. An important life goal!

Key: It must be something that has a lot of POSITIVE emotion connected to it when it comes true!

Step 2: On an index card, you want to glue a small picture or draw one of what you identified in Step 1.

> **Key:** What we really want is a "visual" representation of it so that when you look at the index card, you can immediately feel the emotion you'll have when it comes true!

Step 3: Carry this index card with you wherever you go and be sure to look at it several times a day to keep you focused on *wellness*!

Here is mine:

About 10 years ago I climbed to the top of Half Dome, which is in Yosemite National Park. It has always been my goal to go back ten years later and climb it again! For me, this would be the ultimate proof that I am still in great shape despite being in my 60's!

Bonus Tip:

On the second side I wrote the exact words I wanted to hear from the doctor & would visualize him saying them to me!

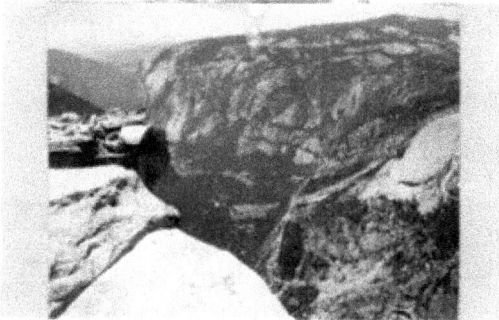

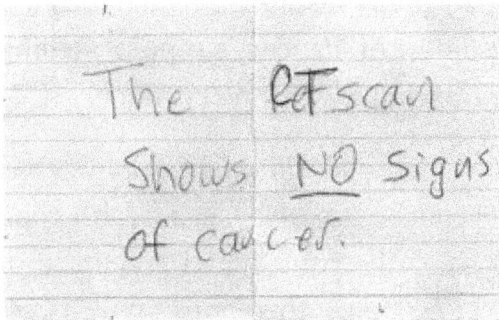

The PET scan Shows NO signs of cancer.

IMPORTANT POINT –
Once you *know* your doctor better, only use the words they would say otherwise your brain may reject it. Mine changed to: ***"Everything looks good. We'll see you in 6 months."***

The Energy Philosophy
Cornerstone #3

This brings us to the next cornerstone in my **Survivor Mindset™** which is *Healing.*

There are two different approaches to cancer people can embrace:

There is the *Fighting Philosophy* which has the focus cancer is something you must beat, conquer, gain power over, or win the fight against. For many decades this tended to be the most popular of cancer support groups and publications and it is still very much.

Then there is the *Healing Philosophy* which has the focus cancer is a disease, a health condition just like any other and when given the proper resources & help, the body will return to homeostasis and health is restored. In the past decade alone, the number of cancer support groups and publications with this focus has grown a great deal.

I think it's vital to point out that both mindsets have nothing to do with the specific treatment route a person chooses. There are many people who have chosen the conventional route of surgery, chemotherapy, and radiation and they embrace the *Healing Philosophy*. Just as there are those who have chosen the alternative route with little to no conventional treatment, and they embrace the *Fighting Philosophy.* There is no right or wrong one! It's about understanding which one works BEST for you!

I made the decision I wanted to focus on healing and not fighting. Afterall, I have spent 30 years in healthcare helping people heal. But my decision goes even deeper than that. From the day I was born, I was exposed to the philosophy of healing through my father's work as a physician.

I remember quite vividly watching people come to see my father back in the late 70's. They'd come in wheelchairs because their arthritis was so bad, they couldn't walk and after 6 months of working with my father, be walking with nothing more than a cane. My father was way ahead of his time! I later learned that his approach to medicine would be described today as a functional medicine.

The other part to my decision is that I looked at both mindsets as an energy exchange as well. How would I prefer to spend my energy? Did I want to spend it "fighting" or did I want to spend it healing? The illustration below shows how I saw the difference between the two. And for me, I choose to spend it healing.

Where Is My Energy Going?

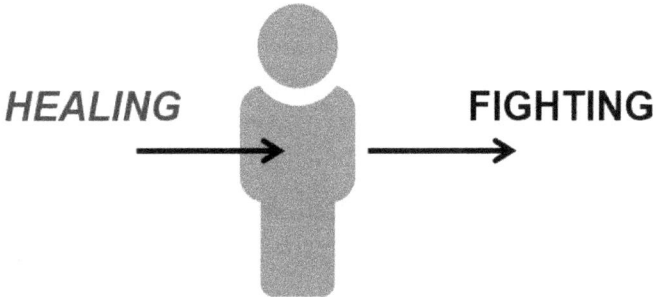

HEALING   FIGHTING

The Acceptance Quotient™
Cornerstone #4

There is one last cornerstone in the **Survivor's Mindset™** which is *Acceptance.*

This will not only determine to what extent you'll be able to truly benefit from this book and use the incredible new tools you're about to learn. It also can influence how you pursue your own road to recovery from cancer.

During my years in clinical practice, I've developed a simple way for people to understand this concept and where they are using the picture below:

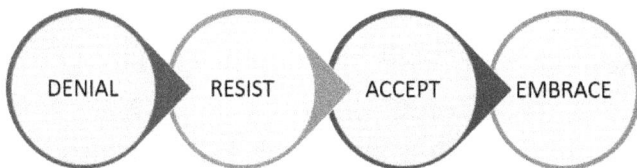

I think it is most helpful to connect these to an example for each stage. The following scenarios are case portrayals I created to help you better understand a person at each stage.

DENIAL

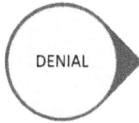

Joe is someone who has a history of a test result showing his PSA was super high, indicating he could have prostate cancer. Normally, the next step would be to do a biopsy. But every time his doctor brought it up, Joe just kept shrugging it off. Joe's wife was very upset because Joe didn't want to talk about it. He was adamant, he was fine and in good health.

RESIST

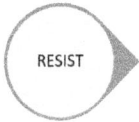

Susan is someone who's been diagnosed with breast cancer but is having a hard time getting to her appointments. She has scheduled the biopsy but also changed it a few times. Her sister is concerned she is dragging her feet following through because she's struggling to fully accept her diagnosis.

ACCEPT

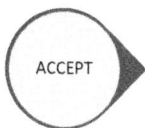

Karen was diagnosed with lung cancer last year and has been working with her naturopathic doctor ever since. While she did have the surgery as was recommended, she did not want to do chemotherapy and radiation. Rather she wanted to pursue a more alternative course of treatment. She had a close friend who had great success working with this doctor and believes she can too.

EMBRACE

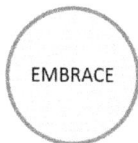

Stan was diagnosed in late-stage pancreatic cancer with metastases to his lungs and told he would only have 1-2 years to live. He realized he needed to completely change the unhealthy lifestyle he'd been living up till now & felt he had been given a "wake up call". He also decided after doing some research, to work with an integrative oncologist. He wanted to be sure he was doing everything he could, traditional and complimentary, to help his body recover.

There were 2 critical points I always tried to communicate to my patients that are just as important for you to understand:

1) Acceptance does not mean "like". We can accept and still not like the fact we have cancer! It means to *see it as it really is.*

2) There is *no one road or path to acceptance.* Each person has their own unique way of arriving where they are. And where you are is where you stay until you change it!

One of the many amazing benefits of being a part of a cancer support group is it can enable you to grow in your level of acceptance. I highly recommend finding a group that fits best with your type of cancer or treatment route.

So, my question for you is this:

Where do you find yourself to currently be in terms of your Acceptance Quotient?

I can tell you where you are not:

You are not at **Denial** if you are still reading this book! Joe would have not even accepted the book in the first place!

Part Two

Taking Control of Stress

Don't Miss Out...

> **A Special Gift**
>
> **Is Waiting**
>
> **Just For You!**

Carol has put together a
special eBook just for you...

To sign up for
"Your C.A.L.M. Toolbox"

Go to:

StandTallToCancer.com

About This Part

I doubt you have read a 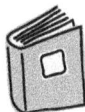 like this!

I like to use a lot of pictures, 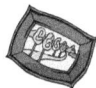 analogies, & word art which help information stick in the brain!

I call my approach:

SMARTheory™

(It's what makes my books and services *different* from all others!)

KNOWLEDGE is the *left brain* at work.

This is where YOU ***know*** what to do!

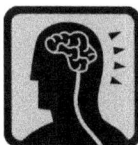

Since I use "pictures" & "images", I end up

tapping into the other side of the brain –

the right side!

With both sides working

on the same page,

the end result is getting people to

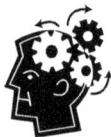

Move knowledge into ACTION

and ***start using what they learn!***

What Is Stress?

STRESS is...

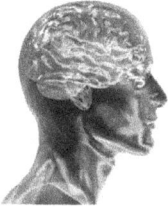

Our
Brain's
Survival
Mechanism

Our brain has one job it is focused on:
Keeping us ALIVE... 24 hours a day!

It is "hardwired" to respond to *any*

Change or Situation

(This means we don't get to control it!)

How many changes or situations do you
face in just one day? A LOT!

It's important to understand
STRESS comes wrapped in a
lot of different packages...

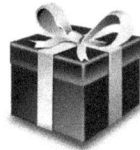

Stress can be...

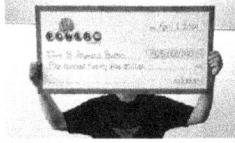

Winning $400 million Powerball!

or

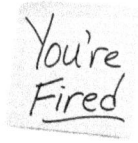

Getting terminated from a job.

It can also be a...

BIG
change

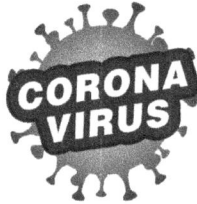

or

SMALL
change

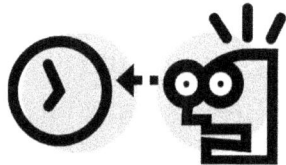

Leaving 5 minutes late!

Our brain has **3 basic responses**

to stress:

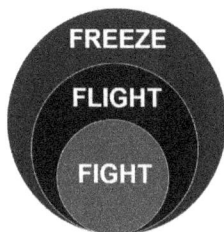

Most people have heard of these before.

But there's one more response I've

discovered during my **30** year career...

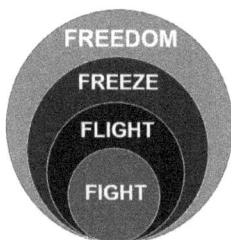

By taking steps to **MANAGE** the responses,

They are no longer negatively impacting us!

The Impact of Stress on Cancer

The research shows…

STRESS has a huge impact on cancer.

MEDICALNEWSTODAY

How chronic stress boosts cancer cell growth

newsmax health

Stress Causes Cancer to Spread Six Times Faster

ScienceDaily

Your source for the latest research news

Stress suppresses response to cancer treatments

Date: November 27, 2017

Source: University of Queensland

So, what does this mean?

Stress *is* a **HUGE** problem

The ? is:

What is stress COSTING YOU?

Are you so stressed out you can't sleep?

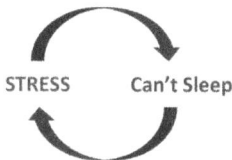

STRESS   Can't Sleep

Is stress spilling out on the wrong people?

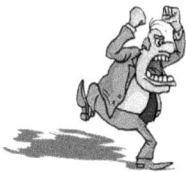

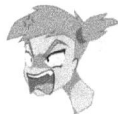

Are you having anxiety or depression??

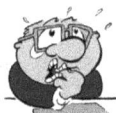

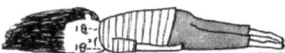

Are more health issues showing up?

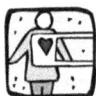

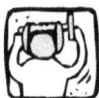

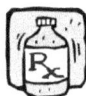

A "yes" to any of these is a sure sign
stress has *taken CONTROL* of your life.

Chances are...

no matter what you've tried it still
DOESN'T HELP.

That's because what *we've been taught* is

ALL WRONG!

Let Me Explain...

I used to get stressed out at work by

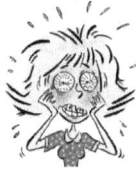

10:00 am

Stress management

meant going to the gym to exercise at

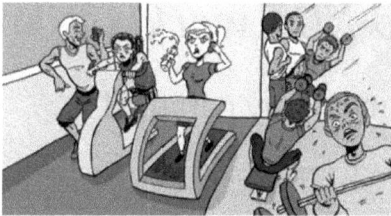

6:00 pm

or

Getting a massage at

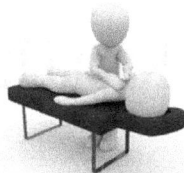

7:00 pm

The **problem** is...

MIGRAINES

would come at

2:00 pm!

I discovered that having to wait

to do a "stress management" activity

did NOT work...

for me or my patients!

This led me to develop a new approach

to dealing with stress & anxiety called:

Rapid Relief Therapy ™

So, what is it?

What Is Rapid Relief Therapy™?

It's when you get stressed out...

at 10:00 am

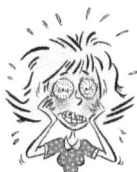

Being able to take
ACTION INSTANTLY
to reduce stress & anxiety!

This is how I got control of my migraines!

Now instead...

60 secs.

MIGRAINE
AVOIDED!

10:02 am

10:00 am

60 secs.

Punching
Bag

There's another way to understand it:

Just like a 🪙 -

STRESS has two sides.

Don't get me wrong!

Stress management has its place in

our lives as a great prevention tool.

However, that's only **1** side.

We need to work on the other side too!

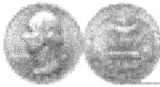

PREVENTION   🪙🪙   **INTERVENTION**

⇓   ⇓

Stress   **Rapid Relief**
Management   **Therapy™**

WE MUST DO & LEARN BOTH!!!!

Tracking Your Progress

I developed a tool to help my patients

be able to track their progress.

The Stressometer™

It's pretty simple to use!

1st - Read each question & select the answer that ***best describes* you.**

2nd - When you get to the end, ***total up*** all the numbers for a score

3rd - ***Check your score*** on the key. Repeat to see how you progress!

The Stressometer™

I find when I try to sleep, my mind just keeps racing about things.

1	2	3	4	5	6	7

Not at all · · · · · · · · · All the time

I find my appetite changes, I'm either eating more or eating less.

1	2	3	4	5	6	7

Not at all · · · · · · · · · All the time

I find myself getting really angry or irritated over the littlest things.

1	2	3	4	5	6	7

Not at all · · · · · · · · · All the time

I find I am having increased health issues. (ie. migraines, pain, & digestive)

1	2	3	4	5	6	7

Not at all · · · · · · · · · All the time

I find my relationships are being impacted by everything going on now in my life.

1	2	3	4	5	6	7

Not at all · · · · · · · · · All the time

Total: _____

How Stressed Are You?

5–10 **Great news!**
You have no stress!

11–15 **Good news!**
You have just a little bit of stress!

16–20 **Not bad!**
You still have a handle on it!

21–25 **WATCH OUT!**
STRESS is *starting to cause trouble!*

26–30 **WARNING...**
STRESS is *greatly impacting* your life.

31–35 **DANGER Zone!**
Your level has you at extreme risk.

Your score ***will come down*** when

you use the system!!!

Use the online version:

StressYOUniversity.com/Stressometer-IANC

Another Tracking Tool

How to tell if this 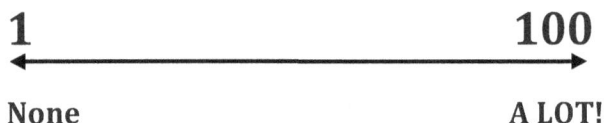 is helping!

There are 2 more ways to track -

Both use a score of 1 to 100

1   **100**

⟵————————————————⟶

None   **A LOT!**

#1 Track your **daily** stress level
(do this every evening)

#2 Track your level **before & after** you use the tools!

**Since this is new for you
it may take a little time for you to
get used to the tools!**

For CALM system to WORK...

YOU must *take* **ACTION!**

Here are a couple of my **WordTools™** to help:

A

Critical

Task

Implemented

Only

Now!

© 2022 & licensed by Well YOUniversity, LLC

Taken from the *WordTools™ Series*

No "tool" will work...

if you don't **pick it up**

&

DO something with it!!

Here's my WordTool™:

D irect

O pportunity

And,

When we **DON'T** use the "tools"

This is what happens!

D enied

O pportunity

N ot

' T rying

Making Stress Visible

What if ...

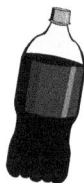

We take a bottle of root beer

and SHAKE it up a lot!

So,

what do you think will **happen**

to the bottle of root beer?

You're **right!**

The PRESSURE will build up inside!

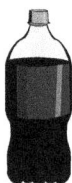 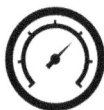

It's same way with stress...

Life happens every day to

shake us up!

And...

Just like the pressure

BUILDS UP

in the bottle...

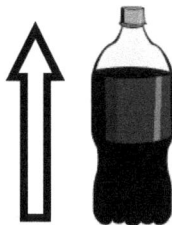

PRESSURE builds up _inside us!_

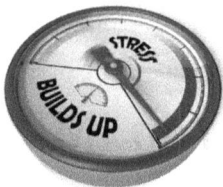

Sometimes it's just _a little pressure_

&

other times _it can be **a lot** of PRESSURE_

Unfortunately,

Most people ***don't recognize***

how much pressure is building up

until it's **too late.**

This leads to one of 2 things happening:

#1 – You EXPLODE

And it comes spilling out

on the wrong people.

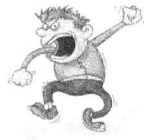

#2 – You IMPLODE

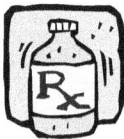
And it stays inside

but makes you sick.

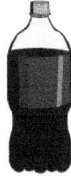

If we look at the bottle of root beer

We *SEE* *the pressure's built up*:

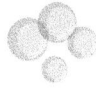

Because the bubbles show up on top.

You must begin to recognize

when the pressure is

building up   in **YOU!**

is going to help you do just that!

The Calm Code™

The framework you're about to discover

has the power to give you

*complete control
over cancer stress & anxiety.*

The 4 steps of the **Calm Code™** are

designed so that each step builds on the last.

```
    Step 1              Step 2
┌──────────────┐    ┌──────────────┐
│ CONNECT      │ ─→ │ AWARE        │
└──────────────┘    └──────────────┘
      ↑                    │
      │                    ↓
┌──────────────┐    ┌──────────────┐
│ MINDFARE     │ ←─ │ LET OUT      │
└──────────────┘    └──────────────┘
    Step 4              Step 3
```

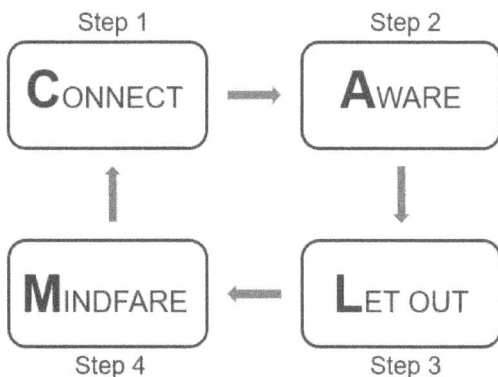

Let's now go through
each one of these steps...

Step 1

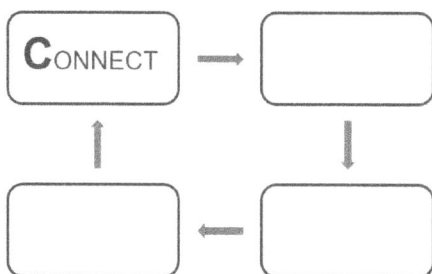

This is the **most important** step - without it, none of the others can be taken!

As soon as my surgery date was set,

I struggled for the next few days.

I couldn't 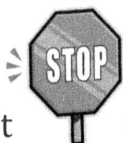 these negative

thoughts from trying to *hijack my brain.*

REMEMBER: We cannot stop our thoughts,
*we can only **manage them!***

The Danger Zones

There were 2 directions these thoughts

would try to take me...

#1

The "Why Me" Detour

#2

"What If" Alley

The problem is...

when we are in one of those places,

We are **not** in the *one place*

we can DO SOMETHING about stress...

the PRESENT!

The "WHY Me" Detour

This is the **first** dangerous place

to get lost in.

Some of my **Why Me's...**

- *Why did this happen to me?*

- *It's not fair… I keep myself healthy.*

- *Why is my family curse haunting me.*

I would get lost in a "Pity Party" –

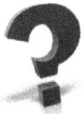

feeling **sorry** for myself & **angry**.

What are some "Why Me's" haunting you?

"What If" Alley

The **other** dangerous place

to get lost in is "what if" alley.

Some of my **What Ifs...**

- *What if I don't survive the surgery?*

- *What if I can't work again?*

- *What if the treatment doesn't work?*

And on & on & on it can go until we end

up so **lost & overwhelmed.**

What are some "What if's" haunting you?

We must stay

CONNECTED to the present *moment*

to manage the stress & anxiety or

IT will **manage** us!

What follows on the next few pages

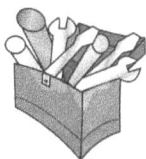 are several tools I use to

STAY CONNECTED.

I want to encourage you to use

several of these tools *daily.*

A little later,

I'll share the *exact routine* I used **every day**

of my cancer journey since my diagnosis!

Connect Tool #1

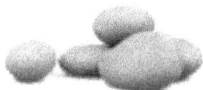

NOW Anchor

1) Find a stone that will fit easily in your pocket.

2) Write the word "NOW" on it with a marker that won't come off.

3) When you find yourself getting "lost" hold the stone & say these words:

Notice

Only

What-is

Taken from the *WordTools Series*

So…

DON'T have access to stones?

No problem!

Here's a **modification** you can use:

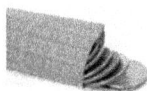

1)   Take a stack of 4 quarters (or nickels)
     & tape them together.

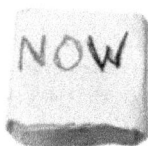

2)   Tape a little piece of paper around it
     & write the word **"NOW"** on it.

3)   When you find yourself getting "lost",
     hold the coins & say the phrase!

And...

Here's 1 more **modification** to use:

1) Take an index card or a little piece of scrap paper.

2) Write the word **"NOW"** on it in really big letters.

3) When you find yourself getting "lost", hold the paper & say the phrase!

* I came up with this card idea for my

patients who'd have a custody hearing...

"anchoring" them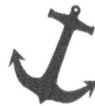

back to our support!

Connect Tool #2

Start paying attention to your:

Thoughts

Feelings

Behaviors

These will be the indicators you're

heading towards **"The Detours".**

When you notice you're getting lost,

say the following phrase to yourself:

'Feel your feet!'

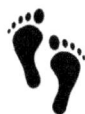

Both tools help ANCHOR you

in the present moment & pull you back

to TODAY!

Connect Tool #3

The last tool I want to share happens to be

the **most powerful** of all!

I must confess...

I first learned it on the job 30 years ago -

But it wasn't until I received it as a

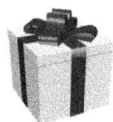

that I was able to **"live"** it:

One Day At A Time

This tool has magic**al** powers!

But,

it's only a *saying* UNTIL it's put into **ACTION**

And this is how you do it...

First, read the following:

YESTERDAY, TODAY, and TOMORROW

There are two days in every week that we need not worry about, two days that must be kept free from fear and apprehension.

One is **<u>YESTERDAY</u>**, with it's mistakes & cares, it's faults & blunders, it's aches & pains. Yesterday has passed, forever beyond our control. All the money in the world cannot bring back yesterday. We cannot undo a single   act we performed. Nor can we erase a single word we've said – Yesterday is gone!

The other day we must not worry about is **<u>TOMORROW</u>**, with it's impossible adversaries, it's burden, it's hopeful promise and poor performance. Tomorrow is beyond our control!

Tomorrow's sun will rise either in splendor or behind a mask of clouds – but it will rise. And until it does, we have no stake in tomorrow, for it is yet unborn.

This leaves only one day – **TODAY**. Any person can fight the battles of just one day. It is only when we add the burdens of yesterday & tomorrow that we break down.

It is not the experience of today that drives people mad—it is the remorse of bitterness for something which happened yesterday, and the dread of what tomorrow may bring.

LET US LIVE ONE DAY AT A TIME!!!!

(Author Unknown)

Second, take a blank sheet of paper &
write Yesterday, Tomorrow, & Today
on it so, it looks like this:

```
Yesterday


Tomorrow


Today
```

Under "Yesterday" –

- Write all the things on your mind
  having to do with the PAST.

This includes *regrets, resentments, hurts,*
the I Shoulda-Coulda-Woulda's, Why me's
& anything else stressing you out.

Under "Tomorrow" -

- Write all the things on your mind having to do with the FUTURE.

This includes *worries, fears, "what-if's",*

uncertainties, I Hope's, wants,

& anything else stressing you out.

Under "TODAY" -

- Look at each item you've written so far & ask yourself this question:

"Can I **DO** *anything* about that **TODAY?"**

If YES - write the **SPECIFIC *ACTION*** you

can *take* under TODAY.

If NO – Just leave it.

There is one last step to take!

- Fold paper back *& forth *just above* **TODAY**, gently rip apart on the fold.

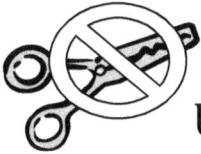

DO NOT USE SCISSORS!!!

It is IMPORTANT to do it by your own hand.

You now have 2 pieces of paper.
Get rid of Yesterday & Tomorrow...
there is *nothing you can do with them!*

Hold on to TODAY

This is the only day

we *CAN* DO anything about!

Do this every morning & carry TODAY with you
thru the day until you're able to live in TODAY!

Step 2

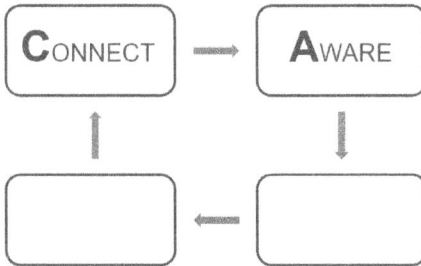

Now let's come back to our bottle of Root Beer with the pressure inside...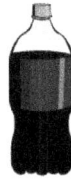

Actively

Work

At

Recognizing

Existence

Becoming **AWARE** means you

now begin to see when the pressure is

BUILDING UP in YOU!

Our brain sends us **Stress Signals**

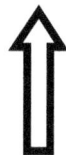

telling us our *stress pressure* is

The problem is most people don't pay

attention to them until it's too late!

Until...

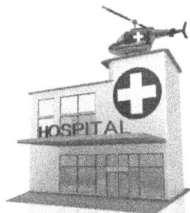

They end up here:

Or here:

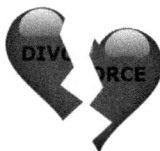

3 Types of Signals

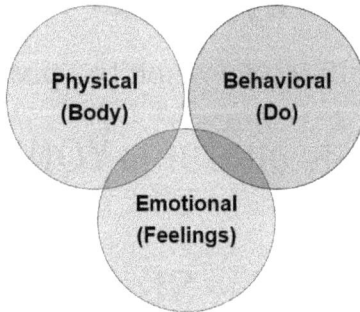

Physical Signals:

These show up in your **body** thru various sensations or bodily functions!

Emotional Signals:

These are all the different *feelings* you begin to experience!

Behavioral Signals:

This is the ways you begin to behave and the actions you **do**!!

What to Watch For

It is **critical** that you start to pay attention

to **HOW** stress shows up in you.

On the next few pages is an **inventory**

to help you begin to ID your

STRESS SIGNALS

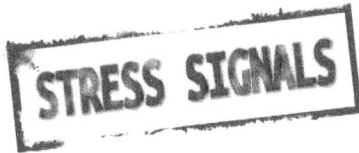

1) Read carefully thru **each** one listed in all 3 categories.

2) If you have experienced, it at *any time* – **circle it!**

3) Be on the **lookout** for when it is building & do Step 3!

Physical: What your **body does**
that you *can't stop.*

Headaches	Tense Muscles
Can't think	Racing Thoughts
Sweaty Palms	Clench Jaw
Feel sick	Food cravings
Crying	Blood pressure ↑
Heart rate ↑	Anxiety
Pain	Confused
Hunger	Can't fall sleep
Tremors/Shake	Diarrhea
Migraines	Upset stomach
Forgetful	GI Problems
Blood Sugar ↑↓	No Appetite
Mind Won't Shut Off	Insomnia

Other: _____

Emotional: What **feelings** you begin to experience.

Angry	Frustrated
Depressed	Defensive
Irritable	Anxious
Worthless	Overwhelmed
Irritable	Annoyed
Pissed Off	Hopeless
Helpless	Jealous
Sad	Upset
Negative	Impulsive
Judgmental	Critical
Impatience	Short tempered
Hurt	Discouraged
Embarrassed	Mad

Other: _____

Behavioral: What you actually begin to **do.**

Eat Junk Food	Shop / Spend
Smoke (or more!)	Argue / Fight
Isolate	Lash Out
Blame Others	Break things
Yell / Scream	Withdraw
Go on the attack	Drink
Self-Harm	Shutdown
Bite Nails	Hold Things In
Verbally abusive	Use Drugs
Avoid	Silent Treatment
Eat More	Sleep More
Become Critical	Get Defensive
↓ Self-Care	Zone Out

Other: _____

The 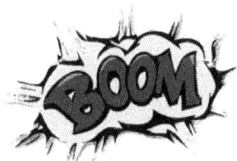 to success...

Recognize your stress levels are rising

&

do something about the pressure

BEFORE you

Explode   or   Implode

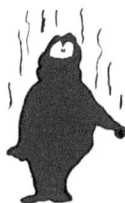

Our body gives us plenty of signals

the level is rising!

Become A Stress Detective!

Has this ever happened to you?

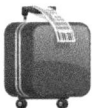 You are going on a trip

the next morning.

You lay down to go
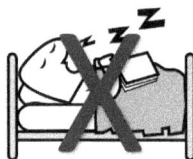
to sleep the night before

AND...

You can't sleep!

This is our "wired" stress response to a

change that is occurring!

Yes...

even ✚ changes can cause

a stress response!

I'm afraid I have some **bad news...**

We can't stop

ALL of our stress responses.

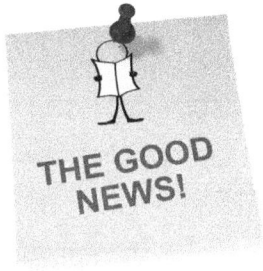

THE GOOD
NEWS!

We **can**

take steps to *minimize*

the response when it happens.

Instead of NO sleep -

I can get *at least 5 hours!*

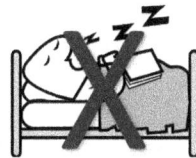

Let's move on to

Step 3...

Step 3

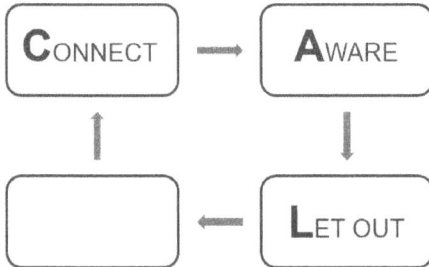

Let's review what we've covered so far:

- Stress = A *wired response* to change

- Impact –It's *critical* we manage stress.

- Step 1 – **CONNECT**
Staying connected to *present moment* is only way to manage stress& anxiety

- Step 2 – **AWARE**
We must focus on noticing the brains *stress signals* it's sending us.

This brings us to Step 3…

Letting It Out

Remember...

Things happen in life that

shake a person up -

Just like the pressure

BUILT UP

in the bottle...

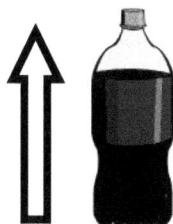

STRESS builds up *inside people!*

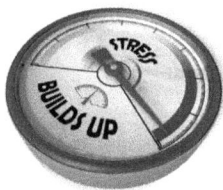

And once the *STRESS gets built up*

It stays there...

It won't go away on its own.

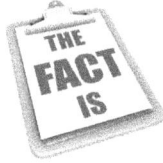

The **STRESS** doesn't go anywhere

Until

we *do something to let it out!*

HOW we do this is

the secret you are about to learn!

And just like the bottle,

It's *not good* for **too much**

STRESS to

build up inside people!

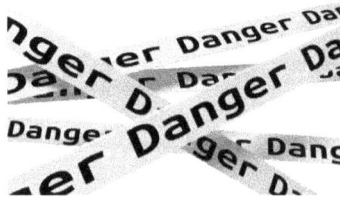

REMINDER: What happens when

TOO MUCH stress builds up...

#1
It comes SPILLING OUT &
leaves a **big** mess.

Have you ever:

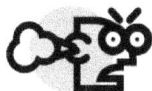

*Said hurtful things or things you wished you
hadn't said, yelled, got in a fight, broke things,
or got in trouble at work or school?*

#2
It STAYS IN and ends up
ruining *your health.*

Have you ever:

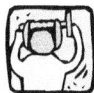

*Felt anxiety, can't sleep, gotten headaches,
ate too much or not at all, felt sad & depressed, gut
issues, couldn't concentrate, worried a lot?*

How I discovered this secret system

was *out of desperation!*

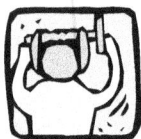 Because stress was

causing my migraines...

I needed to *DO SOMETHING!*

I was desperate....

So,

I started using the "tools" I was

teaching my patients for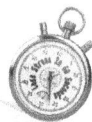

just **60** seconds...

This was the **ONLY** way I could

fit them into my workday!

To my surprise...

it WORKED!

There was *no migraine* that week.

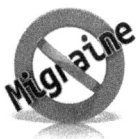

I kept using this strategy &

encouraged my patients *to give it a try.*

Afterall, they'd be more likely to use

the "tools" I was teaching **if**

they **ONLY** had to do it for **a minute.**

And I discovered

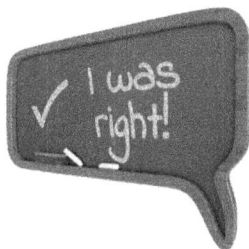

Not only did they report

using the "tools" more **often**, they also felt

in better control of their stress & anxiety!

What you're about to learn

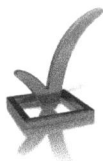

will work for you too!

Over the years of teaching this system,

it has helped **1,000's** of people

just like you **TAKE CONTROL!**

Are you READY?

Let's go...

My Secret System

This is where almost everyone

gets it **wrong!**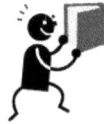

Because you're reading this book...

you'll know the

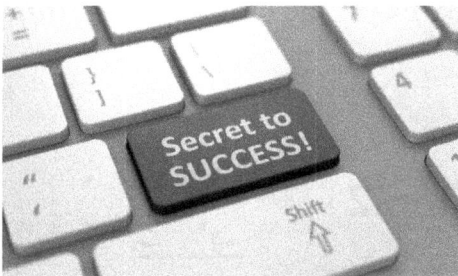

What you are about to learn is *the secret* to

Rapid Relief Therapy™

- ➢ It **doesn't take** a lot of **time**!
- ➢ It will work for **everyone**!
- ➢ It can be used **everywhere**!

There are **2** steps to the

RRT System ™

Step 1 -

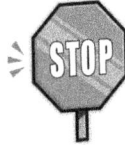

STOP the level from *rising!*

Step 2 -

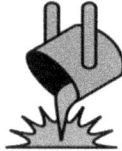

RELEASE so the level *drops!*

Each step must be done *in order...*

Step 1 ➡️ Step 2

Each step must be done *for 60 Secs*

Just so this makes sense…

In order to **STOP** the level from **rising**

you must do something that is

calming for you!

Calming = Activities that require

NO energy or muscles

be used!

I'm afraid I have a little bit of

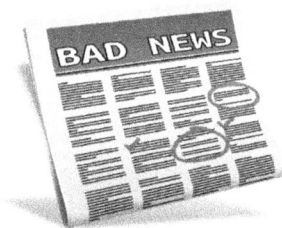

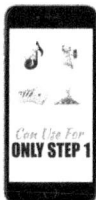

BAD NEWS

You can ***ONLY*** use your cell phone

for this first step!

Cell phones ***DO NOT*** require

enough energy or muscles for Step Two.

Now,

In order to 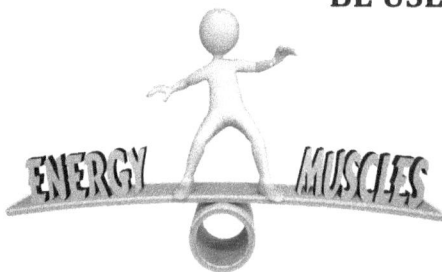**release** & drop levels

you must do something *you like*

and is **active**

Active =   Activities that **DO** require

energy & muscles

BE USED!

So let's apply this

to our stress bottle...

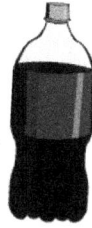

Step 1 - **the pressure**

from continuing to build up!

Step 2 - **the pressure**

that's been built up inside!

Each step:

✓ Must be done **in order**

✓ Must be done for **60 secs.**

** Otherwise the system won't work **

On the following pages are

a bunch of different **"tools"**.

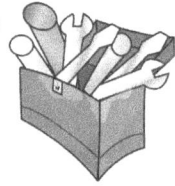

Each one is good to use for

Step 1 -

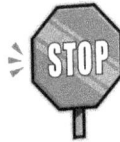

Things from **RISING!**

There are a **4 keys** to

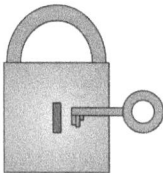

S
U
C
C
E
S
S....

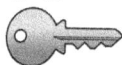

Try out each one.

(***even if*** you don't think

it will work for you!)

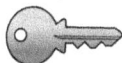

Do 60 Seconds.

(if you can go longer – ***do it!***

30 secs. ***is better than*** none!

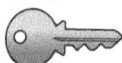

Keep a list.

(write down tools that end

up working ***best for you***)

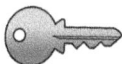

Have more than 1!

(don't set yourself up to fail

the ***more tools*** the better!)

You **must** do **Step 1** *before* Step 2

Step 1 ⟶ Step 2

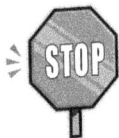 **Tool #1**

read

grab one of your favorite books

Real   or   Kindle

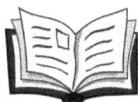   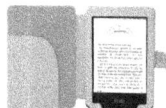

Either way….. you're reading!

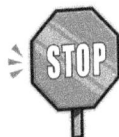 **Tool #2**

Music

Listen to one of your favorites!

Song   or   Artist

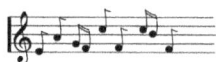   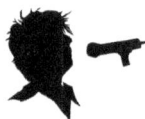

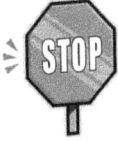

STOP **Tool #3**

Breathe

✓ **Count your breathes**

There are a couple ways to do this:

#1   **Track the # you do in 60 secs.**

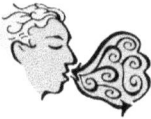

or

#2   **Set a specific # to do 10, 12, 15, 20**

Belly Breathing is best!

This gets lots of oxygen in to our brain...

Oxygen is **kryptonite** to STRESS!

Another way to *BREATHE:*

✓ Square Breathing

1) ***Breathe in*** & count to 4 in your head (1,2,3,4)

2) ***Hold it*** & count to 4 in your head (1,2,3,4)

3) ***Breathe out*** & count to 4 in your head (1,2,3,4)

4) ***Hold it*** & count to 4 in your head (1,2,3,4)

5) ***Repeat!***

Here's what it looks like!

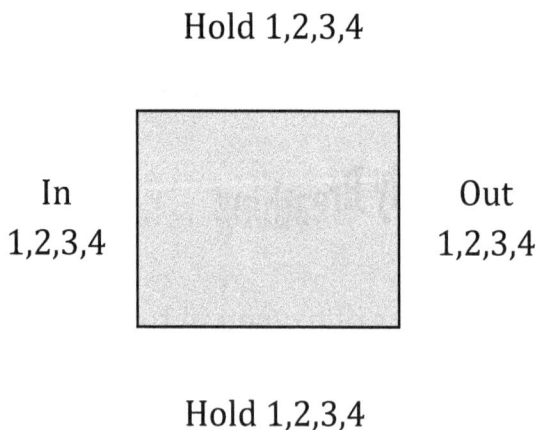

Hold 1,2,3,4

In
1,2,3,4

Out
1,2,3,4

Hold 1,2,3,4

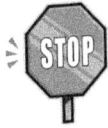 **Tool #4**

Take A Time Out

Remove yourself from the situation.

Create **space** between

YOU & the situation or person

Go outside!

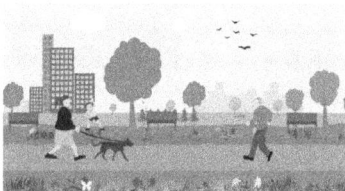

Go to another room

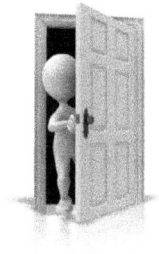

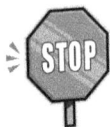

Tool #5

Mind Push Ups!

Here's how:

1. Find a quiet spot to lie down.

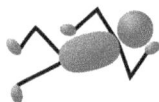

2. Set a timer for 60 secs. (*or more!*)

3. Put a book on your belly.

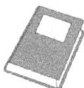

4. As you breathe in, make

   your belly & the book rise up!

5. Breathe out like you're blowing candles.

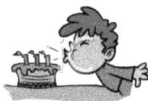

6. Repeat breaths until timer goes off!

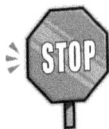

Tool #6

✝ SELF-TALK

Saying positive statements to yourself!

The 2 P's of Self-Talk!

1) Present

FUTURE

I AM.....

THIS IS....

I HAVE....

I will….
I hope…
I'm going to…

2) Positive

~~Don't~~ touch = TOUCH!

Not…
Won't…
Can't…

Our brain filters out the negative
& all we hear is what's after it: **TOUCH!**

** See a list of self-talk ideas on page 104**

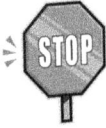 **Tool #7**

The Serenity Prayer

God,

Grant me the **serenity** to accept
the things *I cannot change.*

The **courage** to change the things I *can.*

And the **wisdom** to know *the difference.*

Carol's
'In the Moment Serenity Prayer'

Ask yourself the following **?**

"Can I do anything about IT

RIGHT NOW?"

If yes, ***DO it***!   If NO – ***Let it go!***

Here's a few more *tools –*

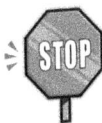

- Guided Imagery on **YouTube**

- Count to 10 **s l o w l y !**

- Watch a favorite show or movie

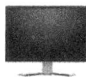

- Blow bubbles

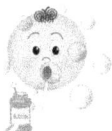

- Lie down & look at the sky

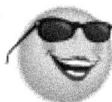

- Picture a sign in your mind

- Make a "Calm Jar" Google It!

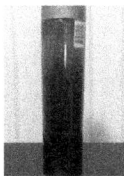

Positive Self-Talk Ideas

I no longer give power to the PAST

Today I feel peace & calm.

I am free of negative feelings.

I am learning to love myself.

Today, I choose a positive attitude.

I am terrific just the way I am!

I have all the time I need.

I am living a healthy life today

Today, I forgive all others and myself.

I am getting better one step at a time!

I am having a great day!

I am a good friend to have!

Can you think of other ways for you to:

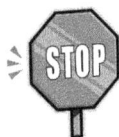

 The level from **RISING!**

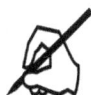

Remember -

This step is one that is calming...

(Requires NO activity or muscles!)

Now we'll take a look at what to

do *AFTER* you have done

Step 1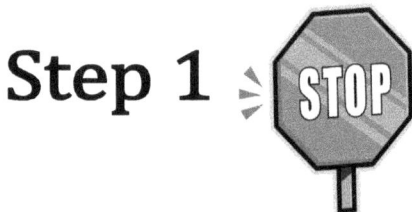

On the following pages are

more **"tools"**...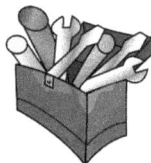

Each one of these is

good to use for

Step 2 -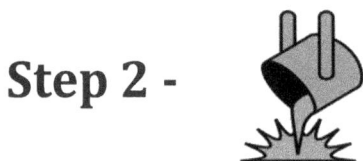

RELEASE what's there!

Again, here are those 🔑 's to success!

#1   **Try out each one.**

(***even if*** you don't think

It will work for you!)

#2   **Do 60 Seconds.**

(if you can go longer – ***do it!***

30 secs. ***is better than*** none!

#3   **Keep a list.**

(write down tools that end

up working ***best for you***)

#4   **Have more than 1!**

(don't set yourself up to fail

the ***more tools*** the better!)

Remember: you **must** do Step 1 ***before*** Step 2

Step 1 ➡ Step 2

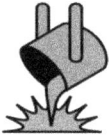

Tool #1

Talk

Grab one of your favorite friends

In-person

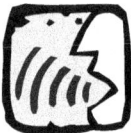

Zoom

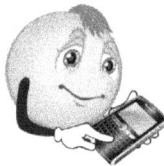

Phone

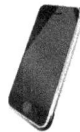

Either way..... You're *talking!*

IMPORTANT:

Talk about your *feelings*, ***not*** the situation!

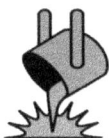

Tool #2

Do A Dump & Destroy

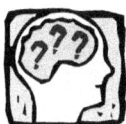

This is one of my secret weapons!

Here's what you need:

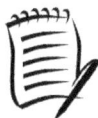

- ✓ A piece of paper
- ✓ Something to write with

1) Start writing

2) *DO NOT* READ IT

3) *Destroy IT!*

It WON'T work with a computer

It requires you to use paper!

This is different from "Journaling"....

with Dumping –

The goal = Just get it out!

Reading IT = *reloads it!*

It also works *really well* when**...

1) You can't **fall asleep**
because your *mind racing*

2) You **wake up** at night &
your mind is racing!

IMPORTANT:

You must go write in *another* room for it to work.

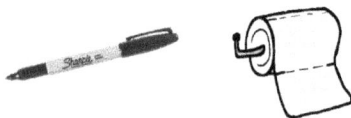

TIP: Use a sharpie & toilet paper, flush
when done. No one will ever read that!

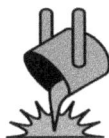

Tool #3

Empty Chair Method

When you don't have anyone

or you can't get a hold of someone

Use this tool!

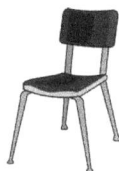

You start talking to the

"Empty Chair"

As if the person was there!

It is a great way to **VENT** without getting

in trouble for what you say!

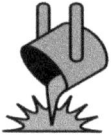 **Tool #4**

Get ACTIVE!

There are many ways to do this!

Walk

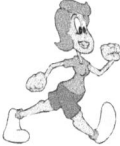

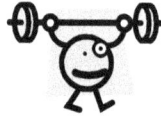

Any Kind of Exercise

Climb the Stairs

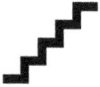

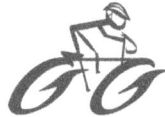

Bike

Push Ups

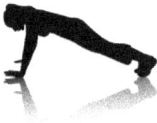

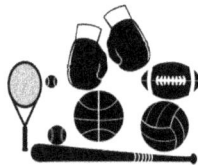

Sports

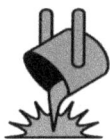

Tool #5

Music

For this tool to work, you MUST:

you **DO more** than just listen!

Dance = Any time you are
moving to music!

sing = Doesn't mean you *can*
or
KNOW the words!

Perform = Play a real **instrument**
or
AIR guitar / drums

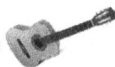

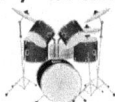

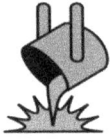 **Tool #6**

Punch n Dump!

There are **2** ways to do this:

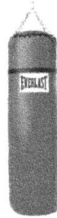

1) Use a real punching bag.

Don't have one?

You can make one using a pillow!

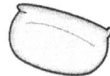 **+** ⌣

2) Air Boxing!

You must ***be sure*** to do this in a

place where it is SAFE.

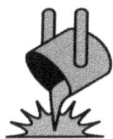 **Tool #7**

Let It Out!

When stress builds up…

Sometimes a good cry or a good laugh

is needed to ***let it out!***

Cry

It's perfectly okay to

let the tears flow.

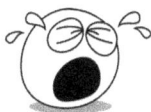 *(Even for guys)*

Laugh

Watch a funny show

Try Laughter Yoga

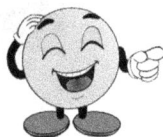

Here's a few more **tools –**

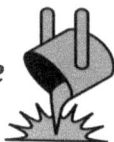

- Tear up an old phone book or a bunch of paper

- Wash the car

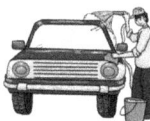

- Do some coloring!

- Rake leaves

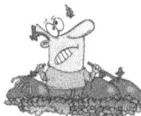

- Do some jumping jacks!

- Scream in a car or another safe place

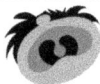

- Constructive Destruction – break something on PURPOSE!

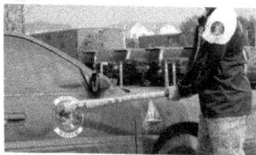

Can you think of other ways for you to:

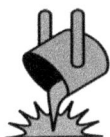

RELEASE what's there!

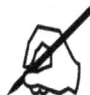

Remember -

This step is one that is active...

(DOES require activity or muscles!)

117

My Daily Routine

Let's face it,

the **stress** of cancer is *ALWAYS* there.

To keep it from *impacting* my recovery,

I knew needed to be

proactive.

So, I picked **5** tools I'd use ***every day***

for at least *60 seconds...*

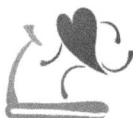
Exercise

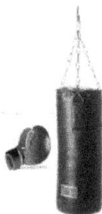
Punch n Dump

Dump & Destroy

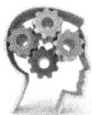
Mind Pushups

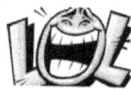
Laughter Minute

I put a checklist on my

& marked it each day!

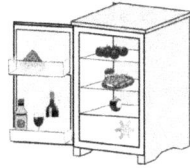

Here's my very first one...

Feb	Exercise	Meditate	Punching	Laughter	Dump
1					
2					
3	✓	✓	✓		✓
4	✓	✓	✓		
5	✓	✓	✓	NYC →	
6	✓	✓	✓		
7	✓	✓	✓		
8	✓	✓	✓		
9	✓	✓	✓		
10	✓		✓		
11	✓				
12	Dr. Cohen / Wappy Left →				
13	✓	✓	✓	✓	

Start is marked beside row 3.

Here's the latest version:

Carol's 5 Minutes To CALM Every Day!

	Day 1	Day 2	Day 3	Day 4	Day 5	Day 6	Day 7
Exercise	✓	✓	✓	✓	✓	✓	✓
Punch n Dump	✓	✓	✓	✓	✓	✓	✓
Mind Push-ups	✓	✓	✓	✓	✓	✓	✓
Dump n Destroy	✓	✓	✓	✓	✓	✓	✓
Laughter	✓	✓	✓	✓	✓	✓	✓

REMEMBER: Before doing anything ACTIVE, you
              must take 5 deep breaths 1st!

Want a copy sent to you weekly to help you stay on track?
Sign Up at StandTallToCancer.com

A Lesson Learned

A few months ago,

I went for bloodwork & something **VERY** *unusual* happened...

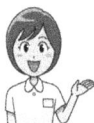

The nurse had an extremely hard time

getting my blood to come out!

Normally I'm a very easy "stick"!

So, she asked if I was under any STRESS

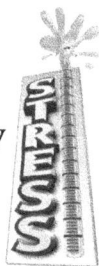

I said *"No, I'm just* **super excited** *about a special project I'm doing this week."*

Then the Ah-Ha hit me!

Even when we **don't** think

we're stressed...

WE ARE!

My body was telling me so.

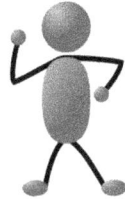

I was doing my **5** tools a day,

but this *wasn't enough* &

I should have been

doing more!

Key takeaway:

When there's more happening in our life,

There's more 'pressure" to manage!

KEY: whether we FEEL it or not...
we must DO more to manage it!

Step 4

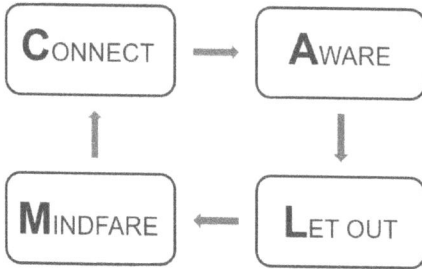

Reaching **freedom from stress**

requires we have a mind that is

working **for us** & *not against us!*

MINDFARE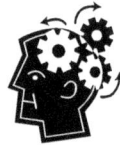

makes sure we are doing just that!

There are many tools we can use

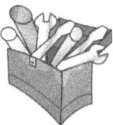 to ensure our success,

let's look at them next...

It's In the Cards!

If you'd come to my live seminars,

as you took your seat, you'd be handed

a playing card!

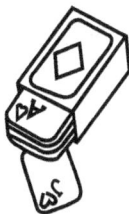

It may be a king, or it may be a three....

The
key point
is:

You **DON'T** get to **CHOOSE**

what card you get!

This applies so wonderfully **to LIFE –**

where we'll face many situations that

WE DON'T GET TO CHOOSE!

This is particularly the case

with a **cancer** diagnosis.

You may have had many plans for how
life was going to go... and now

it changes direction.

However, there are many factors in life

we don't get to control.....

Becoming unemployed

Losing a loved one

Being on lockdown

Health challenges

Buearacracies

So,

what are you supposed to do

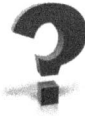

All that you *can* do...

Play the cards you're dealt

the **BEST** that you can!

Here's a couple of the tools I use:

IT'S NOT

WHAT HAPPENS

TO YOU,

BUT

HOW YOU REACT

TO IT

THAT MATTERS

EPICTETUS

Another way to think about it....

We don't get to control the events,

We *do get to control*

<u>our</u> <u>response</u> to them!

We are 100% responsible for our **choice:**

Controlling

How

Our

Intentions

Create

Experience

This is my favorite &

the *MOST* POWERFUL:

WHEN WE FACE A SITUATION

THAT *CANNOT* BE CHANGED

WE ARE **CHALLENGED**

TO

CHANGE OURSELVES

VICTOR FRANKL

Are you trying to change things

you CAN'T CONTROL?

Do the exercise on the next page to see!

127

Write down as many things you can think

of having to do with your life right now:

(Use another piece of paper if you need more room!)

Now go back & circle

ONLY the things **you can control!**

Here's one tool that "makes or *brakes*" it:

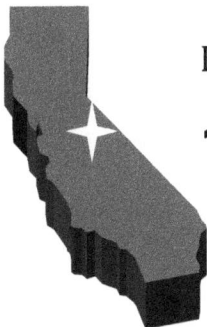

> "Whether you **think you can** or think you can't **you're right**"
>
> Henry Ford

I'd like to share an example of

this quote in *ACTION!*

Ever heard of Yosemite National Park?

I grew up right next to it!

10 years ago, I went back to visit & decided to climb **Half Dome.**

(See on next page!)

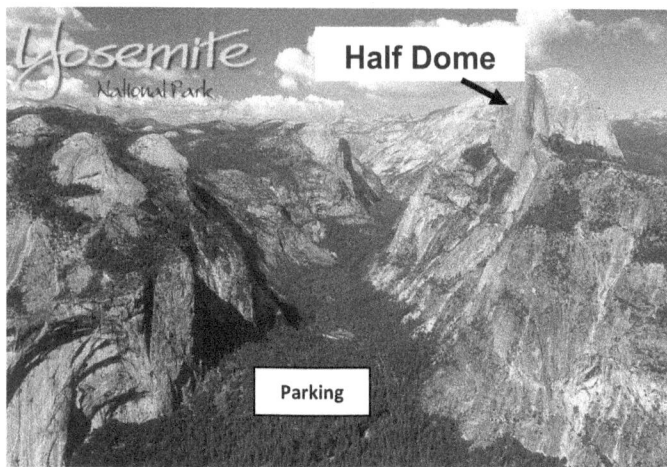

Half Dome

Parking

We left the parking lot at 6:00 am &

didn't get to **The Climb** until 3:00 pm!

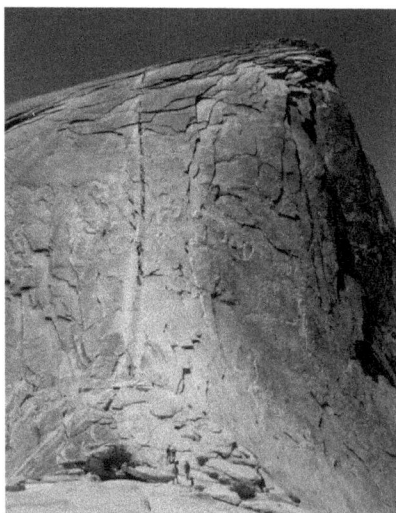

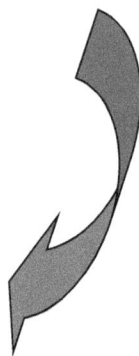

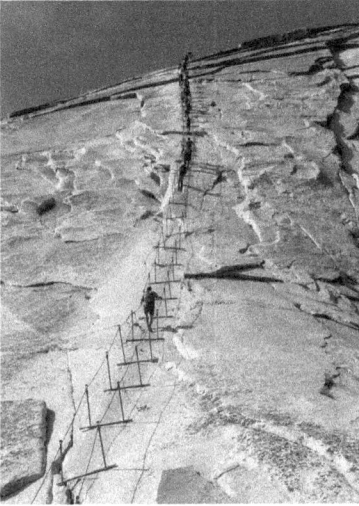

You pull yourself

up using cables!

It's

REALLY STEEP!

My brother & I got separated

from our nieces early in the day...

(They are 20 years younger than us!)

When we reached the climbing part,

I told my brother *"I'm good just waiting at*

the bottom for the girls to return."

I was thinking I CAN'T

Suddenly my nieces showed up

from BEHIND US

& started encouraging us to climb!

That got me thinking...

I CAN

And I did!

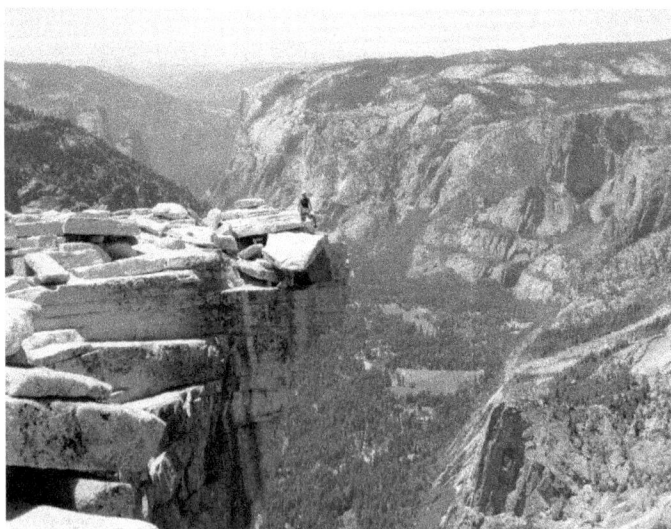

This is the view from the top!

By the way,

My brother was *super happy* to finally

make it back down to the bottom!

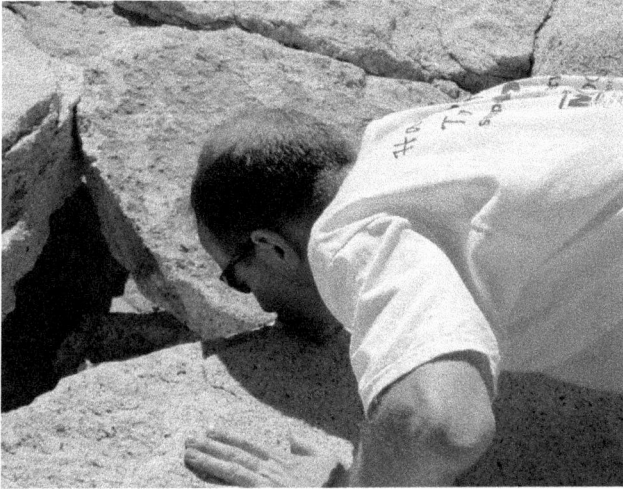

Now,

The ONLY thing that *changed?*

My thinking!

From - **I CAN'T**

To - *I CAN*

Every day we face a **CHOICE:**

CAN   **CAN'T**

(Wellness)   **(Illness)**

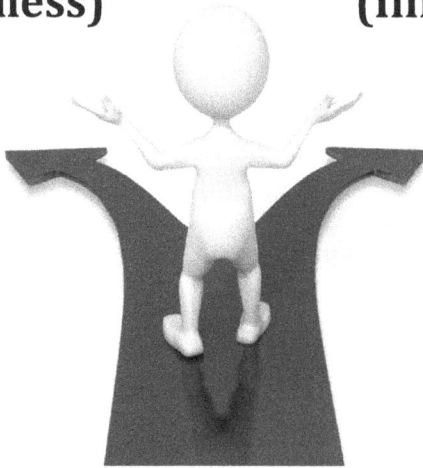

Our Best Health

depends on which one we *choose*!

To *take control* of **STRESS & ANXIETY**

it requires you *choose 'I CAN'!*

The Power Of Mind

Magnificent

Instrument

Needing

Direction

One last tool I'd like to share

is one that helps set the direction

for my mind every day!

Gratitude

Most people are familiar with

keeping a Gratitude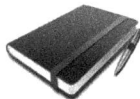

However,

I came up with this for my patients

to take **Gratitude**

to a whole new level!

It's a Gratitude Bank

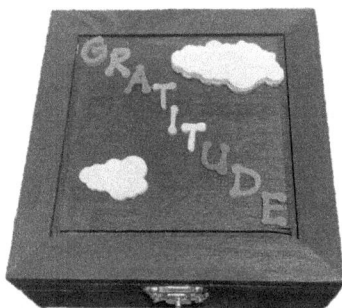

Here's how to make:

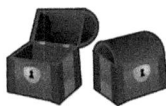

Step 1   Get a little wooden box
(Get a craft store or online)

Step 2   Decorate it as you like!

Step 3   Cut up small strips paper.

Step 4   Each morning pick **3** things
you are grateful for.

Step 5   Write *1 thing on each paper* &
put the papers in box!

Several times throughout the day,

Think about what you put in the box!

The long version

Giving

Respect

And

Thanks

Into

The

Usual

Daily

Experiences

Taken from the *WordTools™ Series*

138

The short version:

Giving

Respect

And

Thanks

Everyday

For

Unbelievable

Life

Taken from the *WordTools™ Series*

So, there you have it!

You now have the power to take

*complete control over cancer
stress & anxiety...*

REMEMBER: The **Calm Code™** is

designed so that each step builds on the last.

```
        Step 1                    Step 2
   ┌─────────────┐          ┌─────────────┐
   │  CONNECT    │  ──→     │  AWARE      │
   └─────────────┘          └─────────────┘
         ↑                        │
         │                        ↓
   ┌─────────────┐          ┌─────────────┐
   │  MINDFARE   │  ←──     │  LET OUT     │
   └─────────────┘          └─────────────┘
        Step 4                    Step 3
```

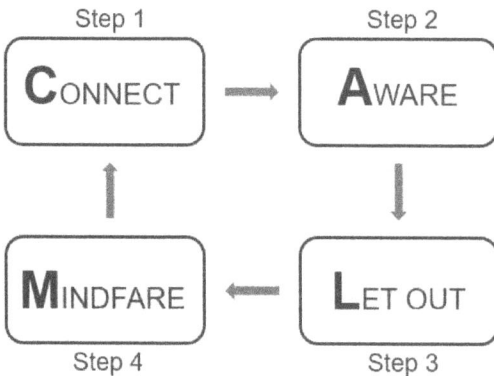

Now it's up to you to...

Put each one of these steps into *ACTION!*

Addendum

I have created a couple of

mini posters!

This way you can rip / cut them
out of the book

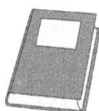

And put them up on your fridge, computer,
or wherever you'll see them!

This will help reinforce the
new tools you're trying to
get good at using!

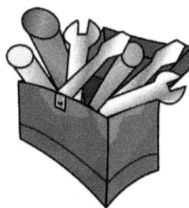

Bonus Tool

I created this tool for my patients &

discovered I **needed** it more!

If you start *feeling overwhelmed,*

I want you to use this:

The Serenity Prayer Stress Tool!

#1 Make a list of ALL the things that are stressing you out.

#2 Using the worksheet on the next page, place the things from your list in the appropriate section.

#3 Fold the paper on the line and **RIP IT IN HALF**. Get rid of what you *CAN'T do anything about!*

The Serenity Prayer Stress Tool!

Grant me the **serenity** to accept the things
I cannot change:

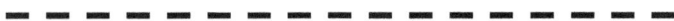

_____

_____

_____

_____

- - - - - - - - - - - - - - - - - -

The **courage** to change the things I can:

_____

_____

_____

_____

And the **wisdom** to know the difference!

RRT System™ -

Step 1 - 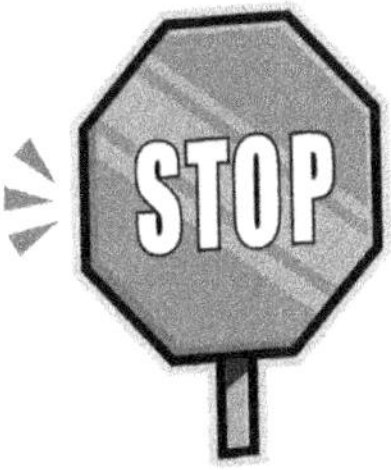

NO
Muscles

STOP the level from *rising!*

Step 2 - 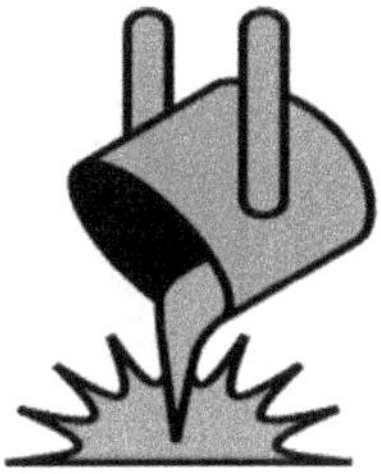

NEEDS
Muscles

RELEASE so the level *drops!*

- **Each step** must be done ***in order...***

Step 1 → Step 2

- **Each step** must be done ***60 Secs...***

The Calm Code™

The 4 steps of the **Calm Code™** are:

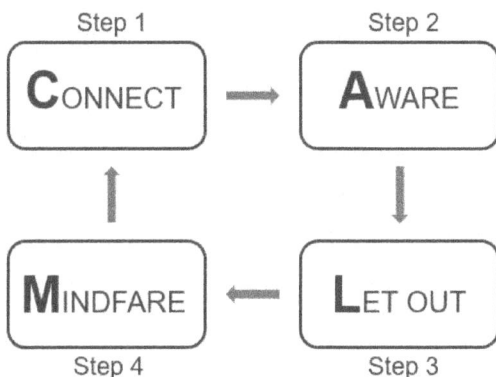

Step 1
CONNECT → **A**WARE Step 2

MINDFARE ← **L**ET OUT

Step 4 Step 3

Step 1 –
Staying connected to ***present moment***

Step 2 –
Focusing on noticing ***stress signals***

Step 3 –
Doing both steps are ***RRT are required***

Step 4 –
Controlling which way ***our mind goes***

The Stressometer™ ⌚

I find when I try to sleep, my mind just keeps racing about things.

1	2	3	4	5	6	7

Not at all · · · · · · · · · · · · · · · · · All the time

I find my appetite changes, I'm either eating more or eating less.

1	2	3	4	5	6	7

Not at all · · · · · · · · · · · · · · · · · All the time

I find myself getting really angry or irritated over the littlest things.

1	2	3	4	5	6	7

Not at all · · · · · · · · · · · · · · · · · All the time

I find I am having increased health issues. (ie. migraines, pain, & digestive)

1	2	3	4	5	6	7

Not at all · · · · · · · · · · · · · · · · · All the time

I find my relationship is being impacted by everything going on now in my life.

1	2	3	4	5	6	7

Not at all · · · · · · · · · · · · · · · · · All the time

Total: _____   **Use key – page 47

Carol's 5 Minutes to CALM Every Day!

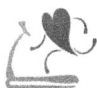

	Day 1	Day 2	Day 3	Day 4	Day 5	Day 6	Day 7
Exercise							

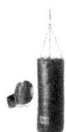

	Day 1	Day 2	Day 3	Day 4	Day 5	Day 6	Day 7
Punch n Dump							

	Day 1	Day 2	Day 3	Day 4	Day 5	Day 6	Day 7
Mind Pushups							

	Day 1	Day 2	Day 3	Day 4	Day 5	Day 6	Day 7
Dump & Destroy							

	Day 1	Day 2	Day 3	Day 4	Day 5	Day 6	Day 7
Laughter Minute							

REMEMBER:

Before doing anything ACTIVE,
you must take 5 deep breaths 1st!

Learning Resources

These are the books Carol read to learn more about cancer & recovery:

Radical Remission by Kelly A. Turner, PhD

Prepare for Surgery, Heal Faster
     by Peggy Huddleston

Beating Cancer with Nutrition
     by Patrick Quillin, PhD, RD, CN

Forks Over Knives: The Plant Based Way To Health by Gene Stone, Editor

The Plant Powered Diet
     by Sharon Palmer, RD

The Miracle of Me by Alicia Bianco

The Power of The Unconscious Mind
     by Joseph Murphy, PhD, DD

How To Starve Cancer by Jane McClelland

Chris Beat Cancer by Chris Wark

Own Your Cancer
     by Peter Edelstein, MD, FACS, FASCRS

The Chemotherapy Survival Guide

   by Judith McKay, RN, OCN

    & Tamera Schacher, RN, OCN, MSN

Life Over Cancer by Keith I Block, MD

The Cancer Revolution

  by Leigh Erin Connealy, MD

The Metabolic Approach to Cancer

  by Dr. Nasha Winters, ND, L.Ac, FABNO

   & Jess Higgins, MNT

** A very important book I had access to:

Naturopathic Oncology

  by Dr. Neil McKinney, BSc, ND

Documentaries watched:

The Game Changers

Heal

Super Juice Me!

Don't Miss Out...

> ## A Special Gift
> ## Is Waiting
> ## Just For You!

Carol has put together a
special eBook just for you...

To sign up for
"Your C.A.L.M. Toolbox"

Go to:

StandTallToCancer.com

Carol's Other Tools

The Nationally Syndicated TV Series:

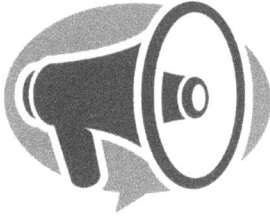

I am NOT Cancer

Watch Episodes at: www.IAmNotCancer.Live

Want More Tools?!

Carol has written other "tool" books!

If you need help:

- ✓ Losing weight
- ✓ Dealing with anger
- ✓ Managing health issues

Take a look at the next few pages…

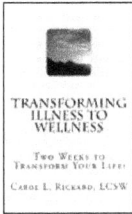

Chronic illness doesn't exclude you from having wellness. Get a blueprint to follow for taking back control of your health!

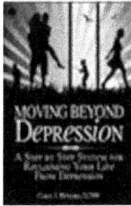

Are you sick & tired of feeling sick & tired? This is a step by step system for reclaiming your life from depression.

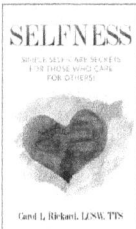

Self-care is often forgotten in this busy world. Carol offers simple and practical strategies to fit in to your busy life!

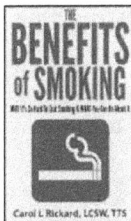

No – this is not promoting smoking! Instead, it provides the knowledge & the 'tools' to finally "Kick Cigarettes Butts"!

Available: amazon.com/author/carolrickard

ANGER

A Simple & Practical Approach for Those Who Need A Better Way of Dealing With It!

Carol Rickard, LCSW, TTS

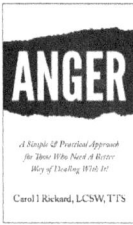

ANGER - one of the most powerful emotions there is. Learn how to manage it instead of it managing you!

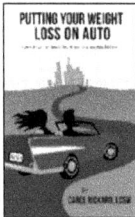

PUTTING YOUR WEIGHT LOSS ON AUTO

Losing weight doesn't have to be complicated! Learn the *7 Laws of Lasting Weight Loss* a car can teach us.
Guaranteed to work!

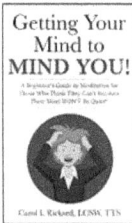

Getting Your Mind to MIND YOU!

Carol L. Rickard, LCSW, TTS

Your mind *is not* supposed to be quiet! Learn how mediation really works & change your life forever!

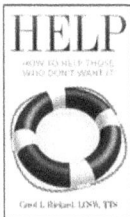

HELP

HOW TO HELP THOSE WHO DON'T WANT IT

Carol L. Rickard, LCSW, TTS

Do you find yourself struggling with what to say or how to help someone you care about? Learn how to say it & what to do!

Available: amazon.com/author/carolrickard

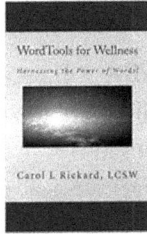

WordTools

What are words tools?
They are acronyms with purpose & meaning!

They are officially called *Artinyms™*, which is Sanskrit for "describe".

On the back of each word tool is a question for you to answer should you choose to!

We have **4 different versions:**

Wellness Vol. 1 & 2,   ***Self-Esteem*** Vol. 1 & 2
Business Vol. 1 & 2,   ***Athletes*** Vol. 1

Examples:

The

Only

Day

Afforded

You!

A

Deliberate

Adjustment

Providing

Transformation

Daringly

Recognize

Experiences

As

Mine

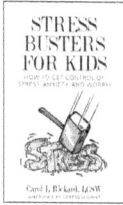

NEW RELEASE!!!!
Kid these days have to deal with so much stress. This makes sure they have the tools to succeed!!

We have three different versions of adult stress books because life circumstances can be different for each.

Choose the one that *best fits* your situation!

Caregiver

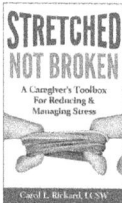

Research has shown caregivers are the MOST vulnerable. Learn quick, simple, practical tools for reducing and managing it.

Stress Eater

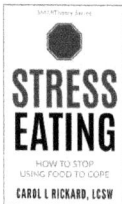

Do you find yourself eating when under stress? Get the tools & knowledge needed to break away from any old habits.

General

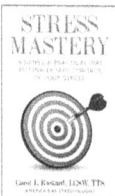

STRESS... It's all around us and NOT getting any less! Get the system Carol has taught to 1,000's & finally take control!

This series of books introduces Carol's proprietary *DO 60 System™* that you learned about in this book! Each version has added chapters geared towards that **specific audience.**

Brides

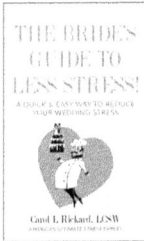

THE BRIDE'S
GUIDE TO
LESS STRESS!
A QUICK & EASY WAY TO REDUCE
YOUR WEDDING STRESS

Carol L. Rickard, LCSW
AMERICA'S ULTIMATE STRESS EXPERT

Nurses

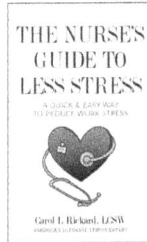

THE NURSE'S
GUIDE TO
LESS STRESS
A QUICK & EASY WAY
TO REDUCE WORK STRESS

Carol L. Rickard, LCSW
AMERICA'S ULTIMATE STRESS EXPERT

Caregiver

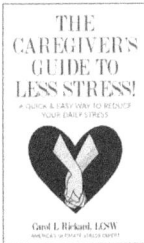

THE
CAREGIVER'S
GUIDE TO
LESS STRESS!
A QUICK & EASY WAY TO REDUCE
YOUR DAILY STRESS

Carol L. Rickard, LCSW
AMERICA'S ULTIMATE STRESS EXPERT

Teachers

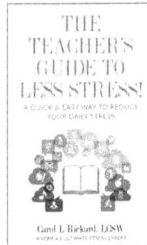

THE
TEACHER'S
GUIDE TO
LESS STRESS!
A QUICK & EASY WAY TO REDUCE
YOUR DAILY STRESS

Carol L. Rickard, LCSW
AMERICA'S ULTIMATE STRESS EXPERT

Available: amazon.com/author/carolrickard

About The Author

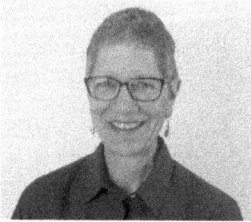

Carol Rickard is a sought-after international speaker and trainer. Her award-winning books and TV show have transformed thousands of lives for the better by teaching real-world solutions for taking control of stress and wellness.

Recognized as one of America's Ultimate Stress Experts, Carol has been teaching stress management in hospitals for nearly 30 years. In addition to the 25+ books published, she has been a featured expert in other publications including Readers Digest, Dr. Oz's The Good Life, and Woman's World Magazine. She wrote a weekly column for Esperanza Magazine's HopeToCope.com.

As a Stage III cancer survivor, Carol knows firsthand the enormous amount of stress that can show up unexpectedly in life and how important it is having the right tools and strategies to help manage stress, so it does not negatively impact your health, your relationships, and living your best life.

She has spoken and conducted trainings for organizations including the NJ State Police, Princeton University, Catholic Charities USA, and US Department of Energy. She was the creator and co-host of a nationally syndicated wellness series called The WELL YOU Show, which is based out of Princeton Community Television. Her new show, *I Am Not Cancer*, inspires, informs, & empowers those whose lives are touched by cancer.

To Contact Carol:

Please feel free to reach out if you have
Any questions or comments. She'd love to
hear how this book has helped you!

Email:

Help@CarolRickard.com

Phone:

US: 888 LifeTools
888 (543-3866)

Outside US: 001 609 462 7643

Want to Speed Up Your Progress?

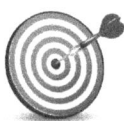

StressMastery
Learn To Take Control Of Stress

You know the **CALM Code**™–

Now it's time to learn the 5 keys to

being an unstoppable Stress Master!

Join Carol for this simple
and powerful online course
which usually sells for $297.00.

Because You're An IANC Reader...

It's Just $47

Sign Up Now!

StressYOUniversity.com/IAmNotCancer